AI-ENHANCED ADAPTIVE WORKOUT PROGRAMS: REVOLUTIONIZING FITNESS

BY

HENRY E. PARKINS

COPYRIGHT PAGE

TABLE OF CONTENTS

INTRODUCTION

In the ever-evolving landscape of fitness and wellness, technology continues to catalyze profound changes, ushering in an era of personalized experiences and optimized outcomes. At the forefront of this transformation stands the integration of artificial intelligence (AI) into adaptive workout programs, heralding a new paradigm in fitness customization and effectiveness. Welcome to "AI-Enhanced Adaptive Workout Programs: Revolutionizing Fitness."

In this groundbreaking book, we embark on a journey to explore the intersection of cutting-edge technology and human performance, delving into the revolutionary potential of AI to redefine how we approach exercise, health, and well-being. As AI permeates every aspect of our lives, its application in fitness stands as a testament to innovation's power to enhance and empower.

The concept of adaptive workout programs powered by AI represents a seismic shift from traditional fitness methodologies. No longer confined by one-size-fits-all approaches, individuals now have access to intelligent systems that dynamically adjust to their unique needs, capabilities, and goals. Through sophisticated algorithms and data analytics, AI not only personalizes workouts but also optimizes them in real-time, fostering greater engagement, efficacy, and sustainability.

In this book, we delve into the science behind AI-driven fitness, unraveling the intricacies of how machine learning algorithms analyze vast datasets to craft tailored workout regimens. We explore the physiological and biomechanical principles underpinning adaptive programming, shedding light on the synergy between human physiology and computational intelligence.

Furthermore, we confront the challenges and opportunities inherent in the integration of AI into fitness. From ethical considerations to privacy concerns, we navigate the complexities of this transformative technology, ensuring that progress remains synonymous with responsibility and accountability.

Through compelling case studies and success stories, we witness firsthand the transformative impact of AI-enhanced workout programs on individuals of all backgrounds and fitness levels. From elite athletes striving for peak performance to novices embarking on their fitness journey, the stories shared in this book attest to the profound and far-reaching implications of personalized fitness.

Moreover, we examine the burgeoning market for AI-driven fitness solutions, charting the course for entrepreneurs, investors, and industry stakeholders alike. As AI continues to reshape the fitness landscape, opportunities abound for innovation, disruption, and growth, propelling the industry into uncharted territories of possibility and potential.

In closing, "AI-Enhanced Adaptive Workout Programs: Revolutionizing Fitness" invites readers to embrace the limitless possibilities of technology in pursuit of holistic health and wellness. As we stand on the precipice of a new era in fitness, let us embark on this journey together, empowered by the transformative promise of AI to redefine what it means to live well, move well, and thrive.

Significance of AI-Enhanced Adaptive Workout Programs

In the landscape of fitness, AI-enhanced adaptive workout programs represent a groundbreaking approach that harnesses the power of artificial intelligence to tailor exercise routines according to individual needs, preferences, and physiological responses. These programs leverage sophisticated algorithms and machine learning techniques to analyze user data, including biometric measurements, performance metrics, and behavioral patterns, in order to dynamically adjust workout regimens in real-time.

The significance of AI-enhanced adaptive workout programs lies in their ability to revolutionize traditional fitness methodologies and address inherent limitations in one-size-fits-all approaches. By personalizing workouts based on individual characteristics such as fitness level, goals, injury history, and even daily fluctuations in energy and motivation, these programs optimize the effectiveness, efficiency, and sustainability of exercise routines.

One of the key advantages of AI-enhanced adaptive workout programs is their capacity to overcome the barriers to engagement and adherence commonly associated with conventional fitness models. By delivering customized experiences that resonate with users on a personal level, these programs foster greater motivation, enjoyment, and commitment to long-term fitness goals.

Moreover, AI-driven fitness solutions hold the promise of democratizing access to high-quality training and guidance, regardless of geographical location, socioeconomic status, or prior experience. Through scalable and accessible platforms, individuals from diverse backgrounds can benefit from personalized coaching, expert guidance, and evidence-based recommendations tailored to their unique needs and preferences.

Furthermore, AI-enhanced adaptive workout programs have the potential to revolutionize the way we understand and optimize human performance. By analyzing vast datasets and identifying patterns, trends, and correlations within individual and collective fitness journeys, AI not only enhances our understanding of human physiology and biomechanics but also enables us to unlock new frontiers in athletic achievement, rehabilitation, and preventive care.

In the context of the broader wellness industry, AI-driven fitness solutions represent a paradigm shift towards holistic health and well-being. By integrating physical activity with data-driven insights, behavioral psychology, and lifestyle coaching, these programs empower individuals to cultivate sustainable habits, improve overall quality of life, and mitigate the risk of chronic diseases and conditions associated with sedentary lifestyles.

How AI is Revolutionizing the Fitness Industry

In "AI-Enhanced Adaptive Workout Programs: Revolutionizing Fitness," we explore the profound impact of artificial intelligence (AI) on reshaping the fitness industry and transforming the way individuals engage with exercise, training, and wellness. As technology continues to permeate every aspect of our lives, AI emerges as a game-changer, offering innovative solutions to longstanding challenges and ushering in a new era of personalized fitness experiences.

At the heart of AI's revolution in the fitness industry lies its capacity to analyze vast amounts of data and extract actionable insights that empower individuals to optimize their workouts, track progress, and achieve their fitness goals more effectively than ever before. Through sophisticated algorithms and machine learning techniques, AI enables the creation of adaptive workout programs that dynamically adjust to users' evolving needs, preferences, and performance metrics in real-time.

One of the key advancements facilitated by AI in fitness is the personalization of workout routines. Traditional fitness programs often adopt a one-size-fits-all approach, overlooking the unique characteristics and requirements of individual users. However, AI-driven platforms leverage user data, including biometric measurements, exercise history, and behavioral patterns, to tailor workouts to each individual's specific goals, abilities, and constraints. This level of customization not only enhances user engagement and motivation but also maximizes the efficiency and effectiveness of training regimens.

Furthermore, AI enhances the accessibility and affordability of fitness solutions by democratizing access to expert guidance, coaching, and feedback. Through virtual personal trainers, interactive apps, and wearable devices equipped with AI capabilities, users can receive real-time guidance, form correction, and performance feedback, regardless of their location or schedule. This democratization of fitness resources empowers individuals from diverse backgrounds to take control of their health and well-being, fostering a culture of inclusivity and empowerment within the fitness community.

Moreover, AI-driven analytics enable insights into trends, patterns, and correlations within fitness data, offering valuable feedback to users, trainers, and fitness professionals alike. By identifying areas for improvement, predicting potential risks, and offering personalized recommendations, AI enhances decision-making processes and facilitates continuous learning and adaptation.

In summary, the integration of AI into the fitness industry represents a transformative shift towards personalized, data-driven, and empowering experiences. As we navigate the complexities of this technological revolution, "AI-Enhanced Adaptive Workout Programs: Revolutionizing Fitness" serves as a guide to understanding the potential, challenges, and opportunities inherent in harnessing the power of AI to redefine how we move, train, and thrive.

The Book's Purpose and Structure

Welcome to "AI-Enhanced Adaptive Workout Programs: Revolutionizing Fitness," a comprehensive exploration of how artificial intelligence is reshaping the landscape of fitness and wellness. In this groundbreaking book, we embark on a journey to uncover the transformative potential of AI-driven technologies in revolutionizing how individuals engage with exercise, training, and overall well-being.

The purpose of this book is twofold: first, to illuminate the profound impact of AI-enhanced adaptive workout programs on the fitness industry, and second, to provide insights, guidance, and inspiration to readers seeking to understand and leverage the power of AI in their fitness journey.

Structured as a roadmap to navigating the intersection of AI and fitness, this book is divided into several key sections, each offering a unique perspective on the evolution, implementation, and implications of AI-driven fitness solutions.

In the opening chapters, we lay the groundwork by defining AI-enhanced adaptive workout programs and elucidating their significance in revolutionizing traditional fitness methodologies. We delve into the science behind AI-driven fitness, exploring the principles of machine learning, data analytics, and personalized programming that underpin these innovative solutions.

Moving forward, we examine the ways in which AI is transforming the fitness industry, from personalized workout routines and virtual coaching to data-driven insights and predictive analytics. Through compelling case studies and real-world examples, we showcase the transformative impact of AI on individuals' fitness journeys, highlighting success stories and lessons learned from athletes, enthusiasts, and beginners alike.

As we navigate the complexities of integrating AI into fitness, we confront the challenges and opportunities inherent in this technological revolution. From ethical considerations and privacy concerns to market trends and investment opportunities, we explore the multifaceted landscape of AI-driven fitness solutions, offering insights and strategies for navigating the evolving industry.

Moreover, this book serves as a call to action for entrepreneurs, innovators, and fitness professionals to embrace the potential of AI in driving positive change and advancing the mission of promoting health and wellness for all. By harnessing the power of technology to personalize, optimize, and democratize fitness experiences, we can empower individuals to live healthier, happier, and more fulfilling lives.

In conclusion, "AI-Enhanced Adaptive Workout Programs: Revolutionizing Fitness" invites readers to embark on a journey of exploration, discovery, and transformation. As we navigate the frontier of AI-driven fitness, let us embrace the possibilities, confront the challenges, and seize the opportunities to redefine how we move, train, and thrive in the digital age.

CHAPTER 1

UNDERSTANDING AI IN FITNESS

Artificial Intelligence (AI) has emerged as a transformative force in the fitness industry, revolutionizing the way individuals engage with exercise, training, and overall wellness. In this chapter, we delve into the fundamental principles of AI and its application in reshaping traditional fitness methodologies.

At its core, AI encompasses a broad spectrum of technologies and techniques aimed at stimulating human-like intelligence in machines. From machine learning algorithms to neural networks and natural language processing, AI enables computers to analyze vast amounts of data, identify patterns, and make informed decisions autonomously.

In the context of fitness, AI serves as a catalyst for innovation, empowering individuals to personalize their workout routines, optimize their performance, and achieve their fitness goals more effectively than ever before. By leveraging data analytics, predictive modeling, and advanced algorithms, AI-driven fitness solutions have the potential to revolutionize the way we understand, approach, and engage with exercise.

One of the key components of AI in fitness is machine learning, a subset of AI that enables computers to learn from data without explicit programming. Through continuous exposure to user data, including biometric measurements, exercise history, and performance metrics, machine learning algorithms can identify patterns, trends, and correlations that inform personalized workout recommendations and adaptive programming.

Furthermore, AI facilitates the integration of real-time feedback and coaching into fitness experiences, enhancing user engagement and motivation. Through interactive apps, wearable devices, and virtual personal trainers equipped with AI capabilities, individuals can receive personalized guidance, form correction, and performance insights tailored to their specific needs and preferences.

Moreover, AI-driven analytics enable insights into trends, patterns, and correlations within fitness data, offering valuable feedback to users, trainers, and fitness professionals alike. By identifying areas for improvement, predicting potential risks, and offering personalized recommendations, AI enhances decision-making processes and facilitates continuous learning and adaptation.

However, the integration of AI into fitness also presents challenges and considerations that must be addressed. From privacy concerns and data security to ethical considerations and algorithmic bias, the responsible development and deployment of AI-driven fitness solutions require careful attention to ensure transparency, accountability, and user trust.

In conclusion, understanding AI in fitness is essential for unlocking the transformative potential of technology to redefine how we move, train, and thrive in the digital age. As we navigate the evolving landscape of AI-driven fitness, let us embrace the possibilities, confront the challenges, and leverage the power of technology to empower individuals to live healthier, happier, and more fulfilling lives.

Historical Context: Evolution of Fitness Programs and Technology

To appreciate the significance of AI-enhanced adaptive workout programs in revolutionizing fitness, it is essential to understand the historical context of the evolution of fitness programs and technology. From ancient civilizations to the modern era, the pursuit of physical fitness and well-being has been intertwined with advancements in science, technology, and cultural practices.

In ancient civilizations such as Greece and Rome, physical fitness was highly valued, with activities such as gymnastics, wrestling, and martial arts forming an integral part of daily life. These early fitness practices focused on cultivating strength, agility, and endurance, often in the context of military training or competitive athletics.

During the Renaissance period, the concept of physical fitness underwent a revival, fueled by renewed interest in classical ideals of athleticism and human anatomy. Figures such as Leonardo da Vinci and Galileo Galilei explored the mechanics of human movement and the principles of biomechanics, laying the groundwork for modern exercise science.

The Industrial Revolution brought about profound changes in society, leading to sedentary lifestyles and rising concerns about the health effects of urbanization and mechanization. In response, the 19th century witnessed the emergence of organized fitness movements and gymnastics programs aimed at promoting physical education and public health.

The early 20th century saw the rise of organized sports, fitness clubs, and exercise equipment, spurred by advancements in technology and increased leisure time. Figures such as Jack LaLanne and Jane Fonda popularized aerobics, strength training, and other forms of exercise through television programs and mass media, shaping the cultural zeitgeist around fitness and wellness.

With the advent of the digital age, fitness programs and technology underwent a paradigm shift, fueled by innovations in computing, telecommunications, and data analytics. The proliferation of personal computers, mobile devices, and wearable sensors democratized access to fitness information, enabling individuals to track their activity levels, monitor their progress, and connect with communities of like-minded enthusiasts.

In recent years, the rise of AI and machine learning has revolutionized the fitness industry, ushering in a new era of personalized, data-driven experiences. AI-enhanced adaptive workout programs leverage sophisticated algorithms and user data to tailor exercise routines, optimize performance, and enhance user engagement and adherence.

As we reflect on the historical evolution of fitness programs and technology, it becomes evident that the quest for physical fitness and well-being is a timeless pursuit deeply rooted in human culture and civilization. With AI-enhanced adaptive workout programs, we stand at the cusp of a new frontier in fitness, where technology empowers individuals to achieve their health and wellness goals with unprecedented precision, efficacy, and personalization.

Introduction to Artificial Intelligence and Machine Learning in Fitness

Welcome to the fascinating intersection of artificial intelligence (AI) and fitness, where cutting-edge technology is transforming the way we approach exercise, training, and well-being. In this chapter, we embark on a journey to explore the revolutionary potential of AI-enhanced adaptive workout programs and their implications for the future of fitness.

Artificial intelligence, often portrayed in popular culture as a realm of science fiction, has emerged as a powerful tool for innovation and optimization across various industries. In fitness, AI represents a paradigm shift, offering personalized, data-driven solutions that cater to individual needs, preferences, and goals like never before.

At the heart of AI lies machine learning, a subset of AI that enables computers to learn from data and improve over time without explicit programming. In the context of fitness, machine learning algorithms analyze vast datasets comprising user biometrics, exercise history, performance metrics, and behavioral patterns to generate actionable insights and recommendations.

The beauty of machine learning lies in its ability to identify patterns, trends, and correlations within complex datasets, uncovering hidden insights that inform personalized workout regimens and adaptive programming. By continuously refining their models based on user feedback and real-world outcomes, machine learning algorithms optimize the effectiveness, efficiency, and sustainability of fitness experiences.

In recent years, the integration of AI and machine learning into fitness has given rise to a new generation of adaptive workout programs that dynamically adjust to users' evolving needs and capabilities. These programs leverage sophisticated algorithms to tailor exercise routines, track progress, and provide real-time feedback and coaching, enhancing user engagement, motivation, and adherence.

Moreover, AI-driven fitness solutions extend beyond individual workouts to encompass holistic approaches to health and wellness. By analyzing lifestyle factors, environmental influences, and biometric data, AI enables users to gain deeper insights into their overall well-being and make informed decisions to improve their quality of life.

However, as with any transformative technology, the integration of AI into fitness also raises ethical, privacy, and security considerations that must be addressed. From data protection and algorithmic bias to user consent and transparency, the responsible development and deployment of AI-driven fitness solutions require careful attention to ensure that innovation is aligned with ethical principles and user trust.

Exploring the Role of Data Analytics in Personalized Fitness Programs

In the pursuit of optimal health and wellness, data analytics emerges as a powerful tool in the arsenal of personalized fitness programs. In this chapter, we delve into the intricate role that data analytics plays in shaping individualized workout regimens, optimizing performance, and driving meaningful outcomes in the realm of fitness.

At its core, data analytics involves the systematic analysis of vast datasets to extract actionable insights, identify patterns, and make informed decisions. In the context of personalized fitness programs, data analytics serves as a cornerstone, enabling trainers, coaches, and users alike to leverage the power of data to enhance training effectiveness, monitor progress, and adapt to changing needs and circumstances.

One of the key benefits of data analytics in personalized fitness programs lies in its capacity to capture and interpret a wide array of biometric measurements, performance metrics, and behavioral patterns. By collecting data from wearable devices, fitness trackers, and other monitoring tools, data analytics provides a comprehensive picture of an individual's physical activity levels, physiological responses, and overall well-being.

Moreover, data analytics empowers users to set personalized fitness goals, track their progress, and make informed decisions about their training routines. Through data visualization tools and interactive dashboards, users gain insights into their performance trends, identify areas for improvement, and stay motivated to achieve their desired outcomes.

Furthermore, data analytics enables trainers and coaches to tailor workout regimens to each individual's unique needs, preferences, and goals. By analyzing historical workout data, identifying performance trends, and understanding user feedback, trainers can design personalized training programs that optimize effectiveness, minimize injury risk, and foster long-term adherence.

In the realm of AI-enhanced adaptive workout programs, data analytics serves as the backbone, powering intelligent algorithms that drive personalized recommendations and adaptive programming. By analyzing user data in real-time, these algorithms dynamically adjust workout intensity, volume, and duration to accommodate individual fitness levels, progress, and recovery needs.

However, the effective implementation of data analytics in personalized fitness programs also raises important considerations around data privacy, security, and ethical use. As custodians of sensitive health data, fitness providers must prioritize user privacy and transparency, ensuring that data collection, storage, and analysis adhere to stringent ethical and regulatory standards.

In conclusion, the role of data analytics in personalized fitness programs is transformative, empowering individuals to optimize their training routines, monitor their progress, and achieve their health and wellness goals with precision and confidence. As we embrace the promise of data-driven fitness solutions, let us recognize the potential of data analytics to revolutionize the way we move, train, and thrive in the digital age.

CHAPTER 2

THE SCIENCE BEHIND ADAPTIVE WORKOUT PROGRAMS

In the quest for optimal fitness and performance, adaptive workout programs stand as a testament to the convergence of scientific principles and technological innovation. In this chapter, we delve into the intricacies of the science behind adaptive workout programs, exploring the biomechanical, physiological, and psychological foundations that underpin their design and effectiveness.

At the core of adaptive workout programs lies the principle of individualization the recognition that each individual possesses unique physiological characteristics, training history, and goals. By tailoring exercise prescriptions to meet the specific needs and capabilities of each individual, adaptive workout programs optimize training effectiveness, minimize injury risk, and enhance overall performance outcomes.

Biomechanics, the study of the mechanical principles governing human movement, forms a critical component of adaptive workout programs. By understanding the biomechanical properties of different exercises, trainers and coaches can design workouts that optimize movement efficiency, minimize joint stress, and maximize muscle activation. Through proper exercise selection, form correction, and progression strategies, adaptive workout programs help individuals achieve optimal movement patterns and mitigate the risk of injury.

Moreover, adaptive workout programs leverage insights from exercise physiology, the study of how the body responds and adapts to physical activity. By incorporating principles such as overload, specificity, and progression, these programs stimulate physiological adaptations that lead to improved fitness levels, strength gains, and endurance capacity. Through carefully structured training protocols, individuals can optimize the balance between training stress and recovery, maximizing the effectiveness of their workouts while minimizing the risk of overtraining and burnout.

Furthermore, adaptive workout programs recognize the importance of psychological factors in shaping training outcomes. From motivation and goal setting to self-efficacy and adherence, psychological variables play a crucial role in determining an individual's commitment to their fitness journey. By incorporating strategies to enhance motivation, foster a growth mindset, and cultivate intrinsic enjoyment in exercise, adaptive workout programs empower individuals to stay engaged, consistent, and resilient in the face of challenges.

In the context of AI-enhanced adaptive workout programs, the science of adaptive programming takes on a new dimension, driven by sophisticated algorithms and data analytics. By analyzing user data, including biometric measurements, performance metrics, and behavioral patterns, AI algorithms dynamically adjust workout parameters to accommodate individual needs, progress, and preferences in real-time. This iterative process of adaptation ensures that workouts remain challenging, engaging, and effective, facilitating continuous improvement and long-term adherence.

Principles of Adaptive Workout Programs

Adaptive workout programs represent a paradigm shift in the realm of fitness, offering personalized, dynamic, and effective training regimens tailored to individual needs, preferences, and goals. In this chapter, we explore the foundational principles that underpin adaptive workout programs, driving their design, implementation, and effectiveness in revolutionizing fitness.

Personalization: At the core of adaptive workout programs lies the principle of personalization. Recognizing that each individual possesses unique physiological characteristics, fitness levels, and goals, adaptive programs tailor exercise prescriptions to meet specific needs and capabilities. By considering factors such as age, fitness history, injury status, and training preferences, adaptive programs optimize training effectiveness and minimize injury risk, ensuring that workouts align with individual objectives and constraints.

Progressive Overload: Progressive overload is a fundamental principle in exercise physiology that forms the cornerstone of adaptive workout programs. The principle states that in order to stimulate physiological adaptations and improve fitness levels, training intensity, volume, or complexity must gradually increase over time. Adaptive programs employ progressive overload strategies to challenge the body's physiological systems, prompting adaptations in strength, endurance, and cardiovascular fitness while minimizing the risk of overtraining and burnout.

Periodization: Periodization is a systematic approach to organizing training cycles and varying exercise stimuli over time to optimize performance outcomes. Adaptive workout programs incorporate periodization principles to manipulate training variables such as intensity, volume, and exercise selection across different phases of the training cycle. By alternating between periods of high-intensity training, active recovery, and deloading, adaptive programs promote

35

continuous improvement, prevent plateaus, and minimize the risk of overuse injuries.

Individualization: Adaptive workout programs prioritize individualization, recognizing that one-size-fits-all approaches to fitness may not be effective or sustainable for all individuals. Through personalized assessments, goal-setting sessions, and ongoing feedback mechanisms, adaptive programs tailor workout prescriptions to match individual preferences, progress, and response to training stimuli. By fostering a sense of ownership and autonomy in the training process, individualization enhances motivation, adherence, and long-term commitment to fitness goals.

Feedback and Adaptation: Feedback and adaptation mechanisms are integral components of adaptive workout programs, facilitating continuous improvement and adjustment based on individual responses to training stimuli. Through real-time performance monitoring, data analytics, and user feedback loops, adaptive programs dynamically adjust workout parameters such as intensity,

volume, and exercise selection to optimize training effectiveness and address individual needs and preferences. By fostering a responsive and iterative approach to training, feedback and adaptation mechanisms enhance user engagement, motivation, and performance outcomes.

How AI Analyzes User Data to Tailor Workouts

In the era of AI-enhanced adaptive workout programs, the integration of artificial intelligence (AI) algorithms has revolutionized how user data is analyzed to personalize and optimize fitness regimens. In this chapter, we explore the sophisticated techniques through which AI harnesses user data to tailor workouts, drive adaptation, and enhance overall fitness outcomes.

Data Collection: The process begins with the collection of user data from various sources, including wearable devices, fitness apps, and online platforms. These data sources capture a wide array of metrics, including biometric measurements, exercise history, performance indicators, and user feedback. Through seamless integration and data synchronization, AI algorithms compile comprehensive profiles of individual users, enabling a holistic understanding of their fitness journey and goals.

Data Analytics: Once collected, user data undergoes rigorous analysis through advanced data analytics techniques. AI algorithms leverage machine learning models, statistical methods, and pattern recognition algorithms to uncover meaningful insights, identify trends, and extract actionable recommendations. By processing large volumes of data in real-time, AI algorithms identify patterns in user behavior, performance trends, and physiological responses, facilitating informed decision-making and personalized recommendations.

Personalized Recommendations: Based on the insights gleaned from data analytics, AI algorithms generate personalized workout recommendations tailored to each individual's unique needs, preferences, and goals. These

recommendations encompass a variety of factors, including exercise intensity, volume, and frequency, duration, and exercise selection. By accounting for individual fitness levels, progress, and recovery capacity, AI algorithms optimize the effectiveness and efficiency of workouts, maximizing performance outcomes while minimizing the risk of injury and overtraining.

Real-time Adaptation: One of the key advantages of AI-enhanced adaptive workout programs is their ability to adapt in real-time based on user feedback and performance metrics. Through continuous monitoring and analysis of user data, AI algorithms dynamically adjust workout parameters to accommodate changes in user preferences, progress, and physiological responses. This real-time adaptation ensures that workouts remain challenging, engaging, and effective, fostering sustained motivation and adherence to fitness goals.

Iterative Improvement: Over time, AI algorithms continuously refine and improve their recommendations through iterative learning and adaptation. By analyzing user outcomes, feedback, and performance trends, AI algorithms identify areas for optimization and adjustment, driving continuous improvement in workout prescriptions and user experiences. This iterative feedback loop ensures that adaptive workout programs evolve with the needs and preferences of individual users, maximizing the efficacy and relevance of fitness interventions.

Incorporating Biomechanics and Physiology in AI-Enhanced Workouts

In the quest for optimal fitness and performance, the integration of biomechanics and physiology into AI-enhanced workouts represents a pivotal advancement in personalized fitness programming. In this chapter, we delve into the symbiotic relationship between biomechanical principles, physiological responses, and AI algorithms, exploring how their integration enhances workout effectiveness, minimizes injury risk, and maximizes performance outcomes.

Biomechanics-Informed Exercise Selection: Biomechanics, the study of the mechanical principles governing human movement, plays a crucial role in guiding exercise selection and technique optimization within AI-enhanced workouts. By understanding the biomechanical properties of different exercises, AI algorithms can recommend movements that minimize joint stress, maximize muscle activation, and optimize movement efficiency. From compound lifts to isolation exercises, biomechanics-informed exercise selection ensures that workouts align with individual biomechanical profiles and movement patterns, enhancing exercise effectiveness and safety.

Form Correction and Technique Optimization: Within AI-enhanced workouts, real-time feedback and form correction mechanisms leverage biomechanical principles to optimize exercise technique and minimize the risk of injury. By analyzing movement patterns and kinematic data captured through wearable devices and motion sensors, AI algorithms can identify deviations from optimal form and provide corrective cues to users in real-time. This proactive approach to form correction not only enhances exercise effectiveness but also mitigates the risk of overuse injuries and movement imbalances, fostering long-term musculoskeletal health and performance.

Physiological Response Monitoring: In addition to biomechanics, AI-enhanced workouts integrate physiological response monitoring to optimize training intensity, volume, and recovery. By analyzing heart rate variability, metabolic responses, and other physiological markers, AI algorithms can gauge the body's adaptive response to training stimuli and adjust workout parameters accordingly. This real-time monitoring enables adaptive programming that maximizes physiological adaptations, minimizes fatigue, and optimizes recovery, ensuring that workouts remain challenging, effective, and sustainable over time.

Individualized Load Prescription: AI-enhanced workouts leverage insights from biomechanics and physiology to prescribe individualized training loads tailored to each user's unique capabilities and goals.

By considering factors such as strength levels, movement proficiency, and recovery capacity, AI algorithms optimize load progression to stimulate muscular adaptations while minimizing the risk of overtraining and injury. This individualized approach to load prescription ensures that workouts are challenging yet manageable, fostering continuous improvement and long-term adherence to fitness goals.

Injury Prevention and Rehabilitation: Beyond performance optimization, the integration of biomechanics and physiology into AI-enhanced workouts enables proactive injury prevention and rehabilitation strategies. By analyzing movement patterns, joint mechanics, and injury risk factors, AI algorithms can identify individuals at heightened risk of injury and prescribe targeted interventions to mitigate risk and enhance musculoskeletal resilience. Moreover, for individuals recovering from injury, AI algorithms can design personalized rehabilitation protocols that optimize tissue healing, restore movement function, and facilitate safe return to activity.

In conclusion, the incorporation of biomechanics and physiology into AI-enhanced workouts represents a transformative approach to personalized fitness programming. By leveraging insights from human movement and physiological responses, AI algorithms optimize exercise selection, technique, and load prescription, enhancing workout effectiveness, safety, and sustainability. As we embrace the promise of AI-enhanced fitness solutions, let us recognize the potential of biomechanics and physiology to revolutionize how we move, train, and thrive in the pursuit of optimal health and performance.

CHAPTER 3

IMPLEMENTATION AND CHALLENGES

Implementing AI-enhanced adaptive workout programs presents both exciting opportunities and significant challenges in the quest to revolutionize fitness. In this chapter, we explore the intricacies of implementing such programs and navigating the obstacles that arise in their development, deployment, and adoption.

Data Integration and Management: One of the primary challenges in implementing AI-enhanced adaptive workout programs lies in data integration and management. These programs rely on vast amounts of user data, including biometric measurements, exercise history, and performance metrics, to generate personalized recommendations and adapt workout regimens. Ensuring seamless data integration across diverse platforms and devices while maintaining data privacy, security, and compliance with regulatory standards poses significant technical and logistical challenges for developers and providers.

Algorithm Development and Validation: Developing and validating AI algorithms for adaptive workout programs requires rigorous testing and validation processes to ensure accuracy, reliability, and effectiveness. AI algorithms must accurately interpret user data, identify meaningful patterns, and generate personalized recommendations that align with individual goals and preferences. Moreover, algorithms must adapt in real-time based on user feedback and performance metrics, enhancing their responsiveness and efficacy in guiding workout programming.

User Engagement and Adoption: Achieving widespread user engagement and adoption presents a critical challenge for AI-enhanced adaptive workout programs. Despite the potential benefits of personalized fitness programming, user adoption rates may vary due to factors such as user interface design, ease of use, and perceived value proposition. Educating users about the benefits of AI-driven

fitness solutions, fostering a sense of trust and transparency in data handling practices, and addressing user concerns about privacy and data security are essential for promoting adoption and retention.

Ethical and Regulatory Considerations:

The integration of AI into fitness raises important ethical and regulatory considerations that must be addressed to ensure responsible development and deployment of adaptive workout programs. Privacy concerns, data security risks, and algorithmic bias are among the key ethical challenges that developers and providers must navigate to earn user trust and maintain regulatory compliance. Moreover, ensuring transparency and accountability in algorithmic decision-making processes, protecting user rights to data ownership and consent, and addressing disparities in access to AI-driven fitness solutions are critical ethical imperatives in the pursuit of equitable and inclusive fitness experiences.

Continuous Innovation and Evolution: The landscape of AI-enhanced adaptive workout programs is dynamic and rapidly evolving, driven by ongoing advancements in technology, science, and user preferences. Staying abreast of emerging trends, integrating user feedback, and embracing a culture of continuous innovation are essential for developers and providers to remain competitive and responsive to evolving user needs and market dynamics. Moreover, fostering collaboration and knowledge sharing among industry stakeholders, researchers, and policymakers can accelerate progress and drive positive change in the fitness ecosystem.

Real-World Examples of AI-Driven Fitness Platforms

In *"AI-Enhanced Adaptive Workout Programs:* Revolutionizing Fitness," we explore real-world examples of AI-driven fitness platforms that exemplify the transformative potential of technology in revolutionizing the fitness industry. These platforms leverage artificial intelligence, machine learning, and data analytics to deliver personalized, data-driven fitness experiences that empower individuals to achieve their health and wellness goals with precision and purpose. Let's delve into some notable examples:

Fitbit: Fitbit, a leading provider of wearable fitness devices, harnesses AI and data analytics to deliver personalized insights and recommendations to users. Through its suite of wearable trackers and companion mobile app, Fitbit collects and analyzes user data, including activity levels, sleep patterns, and heart rate variability, to provide actionable feedback and guidance for improving health and fitness outcomes. Fitbit's AI-driven platform enables users to set personalized goals, track progress, and receive adaptive recommendations tailored to their individual needs and preferences.

Peloton: Peloton revolutionizes the home fitness experience through its AI-driven platform that combines live and on-demand workouts with cutting-edge technology. Peloton's connected fitness equipment, including stationary bikes and treadmills, seamlessly integrates with its immersive workout platform, offering users access to a diverse range of instructor-led classes and training programs. Leveraging AI algorithms, Peloton analyzes user performance data, monitors workout metrics, and adjusts workout intensity and difficulty levels in real-time to optimize the user experience and maximize training effectiveness.

Nike Training Club (NTC): Nike Training Club (NTC) is a popular fitness app that leverages AI and machine learning to deliver personalized workout recommendations and training plans to users worldwide. NTC offers a vast library of guided workouts, training programs, and fitness challenges designed by Nike Master Trainers and elite athletes. Through its adaptive workout platform, NTC tailors exercise routines to match users' fitness levels, goals, and available equipment, providing real-time feedback and motivation to enhance performance and drive results.

Freeletics: Freeletics is an AI-powered fitness app that offers personalized workout plans, coaching, and community support to help users achieve their fitness goals. Using advanced algorithms, Freeletics analyzes user input, performance data, and feedback to generate customized training programs that adapt to individual progress and preferences. Freeletics' virtual coaching platform provides real-time guidance, form correction, and motivation, enabling users to optimize their training experience and overcome barriers to success.

Tempo: Tempo is a next-generation home fitness system that combines AI-powered technology with strength training equipment to deliver immersive and personalized workout experiences. Tempo's interactive workout platform features intelligent sensors, 3D motion tracking, and real-time feedback mechanisms that analyze user form, technique, and performance metrics. By providing personalized recommendations, tracking progress, and offering virtual coaching, Tempo empowers users to achieve their strength and fitness goals with precision and confidence.

Challenges in Integrating AI into Fitness Programs

In "AI-Enhanced Adaptive Workout Programs: Revolutionizing Fitness," we acknowledge the exciting potential of integrating artificial intelligence (AI) into fitness programs. However, this integration also presents several challenges that need to be addressed for successful implementation and adoption. Let's explore some of these challenges:

Data Privacy and Security: One of the foremost challenges in integrating AI into fitness programs revolves around data privacy and security. Fitness programs rely heavily on user data, including biometric measurements, exercise habits, and health information. Ensuring the confidentiality, integrity, and privacy of this sensitive data is paramount to maintaining user trust and compliance with regulatory standards, such as GDPR and HIPAA.

Data Quality and Reliability: AI algorithms require high-quality and reliable data to generate accurate insights and recommendations. However, fitness data can be noisy, incomplete, or subject to biases, affecting the performance and reliability of AI models. Ensuring data integrity, consistency, and relevance through robust data collection, cleaning, and validation processes is essential for enhancing the accuracy and effectiveness of AI-driven fitness programs.

Algorithm Bias and Fairness: AI algorithms may inadvertently perpetuate biases and inequalities present in training data, leading to algorithmic bias and unfair outcomes. In the context of fitness programs, algorithmic bias may manifest in recommendations for certain demographics, exercise preferences, or body types over others. Mitigating algorithmic bias requires careful attention to data representation, model selection, and evaluation metrics to ensure fairness, transparency, and inclusivity in AI-driven fitness solutions.

User Adoption and Engagement: Achieving widespread user adoption and engagement poses a significant challenge for AI-driven fitness programs. Despite the potential benefits of personalized

recommendations and adaptive programming, user acceptance may vary due to factors such as usability, perceived value proposition, and trust in AI technology. Educating users about the benefits of AI-driven fitness solutions, addressing concerns about data privacy and security, and designing intuitive user interfaces are critical for promoting adoption and fostering long-term engagement.

Interpretability and Explainability:

The inherent complexity of AI algorithms may pose challenges in interpreting and explaining their decision-making processes, particularly in the context of fitness programs. Users may be hesitant to trust AI recommendations without understanding the underlying rationale or logic behind them. Enhancing the interpretability and explainability of AI models through transparent documentation, user-friendly interfaces, and educational resources is essential for building trust and confidence in AI-driven fitness solutions.

Regulatory Compliance: AI-driven fitness programs must adhere to regulatory requirements and standards governing data protection, privacy, and ethical use of technology. Navigating the regulatory landscape, ensuring compliance with evolving regulations, and addressing legal and ethical considerations are essential for mitigating risks and liabilities associated with AI integration in fitness programs.

Ethical Considerations and Privacy Concerns in AI-Enhanced Fitness

In "AI-Enhanced Adaptive Workout Programs: Revolutionizing Fitness," it's crucial to address the ethical considerations and privacy concerns inherent in the integration of artificial intelligence (AI) into fitness programs. While AI-driven technologies offer promising opportunities to personalize and optimize fitness experiences, they also raise important ethical and privacy considerations that must be carefully navigated. Let's explore some of these considerations:

Informed Consent: Users must provide informed consent for the collection, processing, and utilization of their personal data within AI-enhanced fitness programs. Transparency about data practices, purposes, and potential risks is essential for ensuring that users understand and consent to how their data will be used to personalize workouts and optimize training outcomes.

Data Privacy and Security: Protecting the privacy and security of user data is paramount in AI-enhanced fitness programs. Fitness apps and platforms collect sensitive information, including biometric data, exercise habits, and health metrics, which must be safeguarded against unauthorized access, data breaches, and misuse. Implementing robust encryption, access controls, and data anonymization techniques can help mitigate privacy and security risks associated with AI-driven fitness solutions.

Algorithmic Bias and Fairness: AI algorithms used in fitness programs may inadvertently perpetuate biases present in training data, leading to unfair or discriminatory outcomes. Biases related to factors such as age, gender, race, or socioeconomic status can influence recommendations for exercise routines, nutritional advice, or health goals. Mitigating algorithmic bias requires ongoing monitoring, evaluation, and adjustment of AI models to ensure fairness, transparency, and inclusivity in fitness programming.

User Autonomy and Empowerment:

AI-enhanced fitness programs should empower users to maintain control over their health and wellness journey. While AI algorithms can provide personalized recommendations and adaptive programming, users should have the autonomy to modify or opt-out of suggested interventions based on their preferences, values, and individual circumstances. Respecting user autonomy and promoting shared decision-making fosters a collaborative and empowering approach to fitness management.

Data Ownership and Consent Withdrawal:

Users should retain ownership and control over their personal data within AI-enhanced fitness programs. Platforms should provide mechanisms for users to access, modify, or delete their data and preferences at any time. Additionally, users should have the option to withdraw consent for data processing and utilization, with clear procedures for discontinuing participation in AI-driven features or services without penalty.

Transparency and Accountability:

Transparency about AI algorithms, data practices, and decision-making processes is essential for building trust and accountability in AI-enhanced fitness programs. Platforms should provide clear explanations of how AI models operate, what data is collected and utilized, and how user preferences and feedback inform personalized recommendations. Establishing transparent communication channels and accountability mechanisms promotes user trust and confidence in AI-driven fitness solutions.

CHAPTER 4

PERSONALIZED FITNESS:THE FUTURE OF WORKOUTS

In the rapidly evolving landscape of fitness, a new era is dawning – one characterized by personalized experiences tailored to individual needs, preferences, and goals. Welcome to the future of workouts, where the convergence of artificial intelligence (AI) and adaptive programming is revolutionizing the way we move, train, and thrive. In this chapter, we embark on a journey into the realm of personalized fitness, exploring how AI-enhanced adaptive workout programs are reshaping the fitness industry and empowering individuals to achieve their health and wellness aspirations with precision and purpose.

The Rise of Personalization: Gone are the days of one-size-fits-all fitness solutions. As technology advances and our understanding of human physiology deepens, there is a growing recognition of the importance of personalized approaches to exercise and training. From tailored workout routines to individualized nutrition plans, personalized fitness acknowledges that no two individuals are alike and that optimal results require personalized interventions that reflect unique needs and circumstances.

The Role of Artificial Intelligence:

At the heart of personalized fitness lies the transformative power of artificial intelligence. AI algorithms analyze vast amounts of user data, including biometric measurements, exercise history, and performance metrics, to generate personalized recommendations and adaptive programming. By leveraging machine learning and data analytics, AI-enhanced workout programs optimize training effectiveness, minimize injury risk, and maximize performance outcomes, ushering in a new era of precision and customization in fitness programming.

Adaptive Workout Programs:

Adaptive workout programs represent the pinnacle of personalized fitness, offering dynamic, data-driven solutions that evolve with the needs and capabilities of individual users. These programs leverage real-time feedback, performance monitoring, and predictive analytics to adjust workout parameters, intensity, and duration based on user progress, preferences, and goals. Whether optimizing resistance training, cardio workouts, or recovery protocols, adaptive programming ensures that workouts remain challenging, engaging, and effective, fostering sustained motivation and adherence to fitness goals.

The Future of Workouts: As we look ahead, the future of workouts is defined by innovation, empowerment, and inclusivity. AI-enhanced adaptive workout programs continue to evolve, incorporating advances in technology, science, and user feedback to deliver personalized fitness experiences that inspire, motivate, and transform lives. From virtual coaching and interactive training platforms to wearable devices and smart gym equipment, the possibilities for personalized fitness are limitless, empowering individuals of all ages, abilities, and backgrounds to unlock their

full potential and thrive in the pursuit of health and wellness.

Advantages of Personalized Fitness Programs

In "AI-Enhanced Adaptive Workout Programs: Revolutionizing Fitness," personalized fitness programs offer a multitude of advantages that revolutionize the way individuals engage with exercise, training, and wellness. Let's explore some of the key benefits:

Optimized Training Outcomes: Personalized fitness programs tailor exercise regimens to match individual needs, preferences, and goals. By considering factors such as fitness level, health status, injury history, and lifestyle constraints, personalized programs optimize training effectiveness, maximize performance outcomes, and minimize the risk of overuse injuries or burnout.

Enhanced Motivation and Adherence: Personalized fitness programs leverage individual preferences, interests, and motivational factors to enhance user engagement and adherence. By aligning workouts with user interests, offering varied and enjoyable activities, and providing real-time feedback and encouragement, personalized programs foster sustained motivation and commitment to fitness goals.

Efficient Use of Time and Resources:
Personalized fitness programs optimize the allocation of time, resources, and energy by focusing on exercises and activities that deliver the greatest impact for each individual. By eliminating inefficiencies and unnecessary activities, personalized programs streamline the workout experience, making it more convenient, manageable, and sustainable for users with busy lifestyles.

Injury Prevention and Risk Management:
Personalized fitness programs incorporate considerations for individual biomechanics, movement patterns, and injury risk factors to minimize the likelihood of exercise-related injuries. By selecting exercises that accommodate specific needs and limitations, providing

form correction and technique guidance, and offering progressive loading protocols, personalized programs promote safe and sustainable training practices.

Continuous Progress Tracking and Feedback:

Personalized fitness programs enable users to track their progress, monitor performance metrics, and receive actionable feedback in real-time. Through data-driven insights, personalized programs identify areas for improvement, celebrate achievements, and adjust workout parameters to facilitate ongoing growth and development, empowering users to achieve their full potential.

Holistic Approach to Health and Wellness:

Personalized fitness programs extend beyond exercise to encompass holistic approaches to health and wellness. By integrating components such as nutrition guidance, stress management techniques, sleep optimization strategies, and mental health support, personalized programs address the multifaceted nature of well-being, empowering users to achieve balance, resilience, and vitality in all aspects of their lives.

Impact on User Motivation and Adherence

In "AI-Enhanced Adaptive Workout Programs: Revolutionizing Fitness," the integration of artificial intelligence (AI) into fitness programs has a profound impact on user motivation and adherence. By leveraging personalized recommendations, real-time feedback, and adaptive programming, AI-enhanced workout programs enhance user engagement, satisfaction, and commitment to fitness goals. Let's explore the key ways in which AI influences user motivation and adherence:

Personalization and Relevance:

AI-enhanced workout programs personalize exercise recommendations and training regimens based on individual preferences, goals, and capabilities. By tailoring workouts to match user interests, fitness levels, and scheduling constraints, AI programs enhance the relevance and alignment of exercises with user needs, fostering a sense of ownership and investment in the training process.

Adaptive Programming and Progress Tracking:

AI algorithms dynamically adjust workout parameters and intensity levels based on user progress, performance metrics, and feedback. By providing adaptive programming that challenges users at their individual skill levels and capabilities, AI programs prevent monotony, promote continuous improvement, and maintain user interest and engagement over time. Additionally, real-time progress tracking allows users to visualize their achievements, set new goals, and celebrate milestones, enhancing motivation and commitment to long-term fitness goals.

Behavioral Reinforcement and Rewards:

AI-enhanced workout programs employ behavioral reinforcement techniques to motivate and incentivize user participation. By incorporating gamification elements, rewards systems, and social incentives, AI programs create a supportive and engaging environment that encourages consistent exercise habits and adherence to workout routines. Positive reinforcement mechanisms, such as virtual badges, achievement milestones, and social recognition, reinforce desired behaviors and foster a sense of accomplishment and camaraderie among users.

Feedback and Performance Monitoring:

AI algorithms provide real-time feedback and performance monitoring to guide users through their workouts and optimize training outcomes. By offering form correction, technique guidance, and performance insights, AI programs empower users to improve their skills, prevent injury, and maximize training effectiveness. Timely feedback enhances user confidence, competence, and self-efficacy, reinforcing positive behaviors and promoting adherence to exercise programs.

Adherence to Individual Preferences and Constraints:

AI-enhanced workout programs accommodate individual preferences, scheduling constraints, and lifestyle factors to enhance user adherence and compliance with fitness goals. By offering flexible workout options, customizable routines, and adaptive scheduling features, AI programs empower users to integrate exercise seamlessly into their daily lives, reducing barriers to participation and promoting sustained engagement with fitness activities.

Potential Societal Implications of Widespread Adoption

In "AI-Enhanced Adaptive Workout Programs: Revolutionizing Fitness," the widespread adoption of AI-enhanced workout programs carries significant societal implications that extend beyond individual health and wellness. As these technologies become integrated into daily life, it is essential to consider their broader impact on society, culture, and the fitness industry. Let's explore some potential societal implications:

Health Inequality and Access Disparities: While AI-enhanced workout

programs offer personalized fitness solutions, access to these technologies may exacerbate existing health inequalities and disparities. Individuals with limited access to technology, internet connectivity, or financial resources may face barriers to accessing AI-driven fitness platforms, widening the gap in health outcomes between socioeconomically advantaged and disadvantaged populations.

Data Privacy and Security Concerns:

The widespread adoption of AI-enhanced fitness programs raises concerns about data privacy, security, and ownership. As users generate vast amounts of personal health data through wearable devices, fitness apps, and online platforms, safeguarding this sensitive information against unauthorized access, data breaches, and misuse becomes paramount. Ensuring robust data protection measures, transparency in data practices, and user control over personal data are essential for addressing privacy concerns and fostering trust in AI-driven fitness solutions.

Ethical Use of AI Algorithms:

The ethical use of AI algorithms in fitness programs requires careful consideration of issues such as algorithmic bias, fairness, and transparency. AI algorithms may inadvertently perpetuate biases present in training data, leading to unfair or discriminatory outcomes in exercise recommendations, performance evaluations, or goal setting. Mitigating algorithmic bias, promoting transparency in decision-making processes, and fostering inclusivity and diversity in AI models are essential for ensuring equitable access to personalized fitness solutions.

Cultural and Social Implications:

The integration of AI into fitness programs may influence cultural attitudes, social norms, and perceptions of health and wellness. As individuals rely increasingly on technology for exercise guidance and motivation, traditional forms of physical activity, social interaction, and community engagement may evolve or diminish in significance. Balancing the benefits of technology-driven fitness solutions with the preservation of cultural values, social connections, and embodied experiences is

70

critical for promoting holistic well-being and societal cohesion.

Industry Disruption and Professional Roles: The widespread adoption of AI-enhanced fitness programs may disrupt traditional fitness industry paradigms and professional roles. Personal trainers, fitness coaches, and exercise physiologists may need to adapt their skills, knowledge, and service offerings to complement AI-driven technologies and meet evolving consumer demands. Embracing interdisciplinary collaboration, lifelong learning, and ethical practice standards can help fitness professionals navigate the changing landscape of the fitness industry and remain relevant in a technology-driven era.

Potential Societal Implications of Widespread Adoption

In "AI-Enhanced Adaptive Workout Programs: Revolutionizing Fitness," the widespread adoption of AI-enhanced fitness programs carries significant societal implications that extend beyond individual health and well-being. As these technologies become increasingly integrated into daily life, it is crucial to consider their broader impact on society, culture, and the fitness industry. Here are some potential societal implications to explore:

Health Disparities and Accessibility:

While AI-enhanced fitness programs offer personalized solutions, access to these technologies may exacerbate health disparities. Individuals without access to technology or who belong to marginalized communities may face barriers in accessing AI-driven fitness platforms. This can widen the gap in health outcomes between different socioeconomic groups, creating disparities in fitness levels and overall health.

Data Privacy and Security Concerns:

The widespread adoption of AI in fitness raises concerns about data privacy and security. Fitness apps and devices collect vast amounts of personal health data, including biometric measurements and exercise habits.

Protecting this sensitive information from breaches and misuse is critical to maintaining user trust. Stricter regulations and robust security measures are necessary to safeguard user privacy in the era of AI-enhanced fitness.

Ethical Use of AI Algorithms:

Ethical considerations surround the use of AI algorithms in fitness programs. These algorithms may perpetuate biases present in training data, leading to unfair outcomes or discrimination in exercise recommendations. Ensuring algorithmic fairness, transparency, and accountability is essential to prevent unintended consequences and promote inclusivity in AI-driven fitness solutions.

Cultural Shifts and Social Norms:

The integration of AI into fitness may influence cultural attitudes and social norms surrounding exercise and wellness. As technology becomes more prevalent in fitness routines, traditional forms of physical activity and social interaction may evolve or diminish. Balancing the benefits of technology-driven fitness with cultural values and social connections is crucial to maintaining holistic well-being in society.

Industry Disruption and Employment Impact:

The rise of AI in fitness could disrupt traditional roles within the fitness industry. Personal trainers, fitness instructors, and wellness coaches may need to adapt their skills and services to complement AI-driven technologies. This could lead to shifts in employment patterns and the emergence of new roles focused on technology integration and user support within the fitness sector.

Education and Digital Literacy:

Widespread adoption of AI-enhanced fitness programs highlights the need for education and digital literacy initiatives. Users must understand how AI algorithms work, how their data is used, and the potential implications for their privacy and well-being. Promoting digital literacy and providing accessible resources can empower individuals to make informed decisions about their fitness journey in the digital age.

CHAPTER 5

THE BUSINESS OF AI IN FITNESS

In "AI-Enhanced Adaptive Workout Programs: Revolutionizing Fitness," exploring the business aspects of AI in the fitness industry reveals a landscape marked by innovation, competition, and opportunities for growth. The integration of artificial intelligence (AI) into fitness programs has opened new avenues for business development, customer engagement, and market differentiation. Here's an analysis of the business dynamics surrounding AI in fitness:

Market Landscape and Competitive Dynamics:

The fitness industry is characterized by a diverse ecosystem of players, including gyms, health clubs, boutique studios, wearable technology companies, and digital fitness platforms. The emergence of AI-driven fitness solutions has intensified competition and reshaped market dynamics, with established players and startups vying for market share and mindshare. Understanding market trends, consumer preferences, and competitive positioning is essential for navigating the evolving landscape of AI in fitness.

Value Proposition and Differentiation: AI-enhanced workout programs offer unique value propositions centered around personalization, convenience, and effectiveness. By leveraging AI algorithms to analyze user data, tailor exercise regimens, and provide real-time feedback, fitness companies can differentiate their offerings and enhance the user experience. Articulating a compelling value proposition that resonates with target audiences is critical for capturing market share and driving customer engagement in the competitive fitness landscape.

Monetization Models and Revenue Streams: Monetizing AI-enhanced fitness programs involves exploring various revenue streams, including subscription models, freemium offerings, in-app purchases, and premium features. Subscription-based pricing

structures offer recurring revenue streams and encourage long-term user engagement, while in-app purchases and premium upgrades provide opportunities for upselling and monetizing value-added services. Understanding user preferences, pricing sensitivity, and willingness to pay is key to optimizing monetization strategies and maximizing revenue potential.

Partnerships and Ecosystem Integration:

Collaborating with strategic partners and integrating with complementary ecosystems can enhance the value proposition and scalability of AI-driven fitness solutions. Partnerships with wearable device manufacturers, health insurers, corporate wellness programs, and fitness influencers can extend reach, drive user acquisition, and unlock new revenue opportunities. Leveraging synergies and complementary resources within the broader fitness ecosystem fosters innovation and accelerates market penetration for AI-driven fitness platforms.

Regulatory Compliance and Ethical Considerations:

Navigating regulatory frameworks and addressing

ethical considerations are integral aspects of doing business in the AI-driven fitness industry. Compliance with data protection regulations, such as GDPR and HIPAA, is essential for safeguarding user privacy and mitigating legal risks associated with data processing and utilization. Upholding ethical standards, transparency in data practices, and user consent principles are foundational pillars of responsible AI deployment in fitness programming.

Investment and Innovation: The convergence of AI and fitness has attracted significant investment and fuelled innovation in the industry. Venture capital firms, private equity investors, and corporate backers are actively funding startups and emerging players in the AI-driven fitness space, driving product development, market expansion, and technological advancement. Embracing a culture of innovation, experimentation, and agility enables fitness companies to stay ahead of the curve and capitalize on emerging opportunities in the rapidly evolving landscape of AI-enhanced fitness.

Market Trends and Investment Opportunities in AI-Driven Fitness Startups

In "AI-Enhanced Adaptive Workout Programs: Revolutionizing Fitness," analyzing market trends and investment opportunities in AI-driven fitness startups sheds light on the evolving landscape of the fitness industry and the transformative potential of technology. Here are some key trends and investment opportunities highlighted in the book:

Rapid Growth of the Digital Fitness Market: The digital fitness market is experiencing rapid growth, fueled by increasing consumer demand for personalized, convenient, and accessible workout solutions. AI-driven fitness startups are capitalizing on this trend by offering innovative platforms and services that leverage artificial intelligence to optimize training outcomes, enhance user engagement, and differentiate themselves in the crowded fitness landscape.

Expansion of Wearable Technology and Health Monitoring Devices: Wearable technology and health monitoring devices play a central role in the AI-driven fitness ecosystem, enabling users to track performance metrics, monitor biometric data, and receive real-time feedback during workouts. Investment opportunities abound in startups developing wearable devices with advanced sensors, AI algorithms, and predictive analytics capabilities to deliver personalized insights and actionable recommendations to users.

Integration of Virtual Reality (VR) and Augmented Reality (AR) Technologies: Virtual reality (VR) and augmented reality (AR) technologies are transforming the fitness experience by immersing users in immersive workout environments, gamified training scenarios, and interactive coaching sessions. AI-driven fitness startups are harnessing the power of VR and AR to enhance user engagement, motivation, and adherence, creating immersive workout experiences that blur the lines between physical and digital realities.

Emergence of AI-Powered Personalized Nutrition Solutions:

Nutrition plays a critical role in optimizing fitness outcomes and supporting overall health and well-being. AI-driven fitness startups are developing personalized nutrition solutions that leverage machine learning algorithms, genetic profiling, and dietary analysis tools to deliver tailored meal plans, recipe recommendations, and nutritional guidance to users. Investment opportunities exist in startups leveraging AI to disrupt the traditional nutrition industry and address evolving consumer preferences for personalized dietary solutions.

Corporate Wellness Programs and Employer-Sponsored Fitness Initiatives:

Corporate wellness programs and employer-sponsored fitness initiatives are gaining traction as organizations recognize the importance of employee health and well-being in driving productivity, morale, and retention. AI-driven fitness startups are partnering with employers to deliver customized wellness solutions, employee engagement platforms, and virtual fitness challenges that promote a culture of health and resilience in the workplace. Investment opportunities abound in startups targeting the corporate wellness market and offering scalable, data-driven solutions to address the evolving needs of employers and employees alike.

Focus on Data Privacy, Security, and Ethical Use of AI:

As the adoption of AI-driven fitness solutions accelerates, investors are increasingly scrutinizing startups' approaches to data privacy, security, and ethical use of AI. Startups that prioritize user privacy, transparency, and ethical principles in data processing and algorithmic decision-making are well-positioned to build trust, mitigate regulatory risks, and differentiate themselves in a competitive market landscape.

Future Projections for the Growth of AI-Enhanced Fitness Services

In "AI-Enhanced Adaptive Workout Programs: Revolutionizing Fitness," future projections for the growth of AI-enhanced fitness services reveal a landscape defined by innovation, integration, and widespread adoption of technology-driven solutions. As artificial intelligence continues to evolve and permeate every aspect of the fitness industry, the trajectory of AI-enhanced fitness services is poised for exponential growth. Here are some future projections for the expansion and evolution of AI-driven fitness services:

Acceleration of Adoption Rates:

The adoption of AI-enhanced fitness services is expected to accelerate rapidly as consumers increasingly embrace technology-driven solutions to optimize their health and wellness routines. As awareness of the benefits of AI in fitness grows and the accessibility of digital platforms expands, adoption rates are projected to soar across diverse

83

demographic segments, including athletes, fitness enthusiasts, beginners, and individuals with specific health conditions.

Proliferation of Personalization:

Personalization will emerge as a cornerstone of AI-enhanced fitness services, with algorithms leveraging user data to tailor workouts, nutrition plans, and wellness recommendations to individual preferences, goals, and physiological profiles. As AI algorithms become more sophisticated and granular in their analysis of user data, the level of personalization offered by fitness platforms will continue to deepen, driving engagement, satisfaction, and long-term adherence to fitness goals.

Integration with Wearable Technology:

The integration of AI-enhanced fitness services with wearable technology will become increasingly seamless, with wearable devices serving as data collection hubs and real-time feedback mechanisms for users. As wearable technology evolves to incorporate advanced sensors, biometric monitoring capabilities, and AI-driven analytics, the synergy between wearable devices and fitness platforms will empower users to track performance metrics, monitor health indicators, and optimize training outcomes with unprecedented precision and insight.

Expansion into Corporate Wellness Programs: AI-enhanced fitness services will expand into corporate wellness programs and employer-sponsored initiatives as organizations prioritize employee health and well-being. By offering scalable, data-driven solutions that promote physical activity, stress management, and work-life balance, AI-driven fitness platforms will become integral components of corporate wellness strategies, driving employee engagement, productivity, and retention in the workplace.

Global Market Penetration: AI-enhanced fitness services will penetrate global markets, transcending geographical boundaries and cultural barriers to reach individuals around the world. As digital connectivity expands and smartphone penetration increases in emerging markets, the accessibility of AI-driven fitness solutions will democratize access to health and wellness resources, empowering individuals of all backgrounds to pursue healthier, more active lifestyles with confidence and convenience.

Innovation in Virtual Fitness Experiences: Innovation in virtual fitness experiences will redefine the way individuals engage with exercise, blurring the lines between physical and digital environments. AI-driven virtual reality (VR) and augmented reality (AR) technologies will enable users to immerse themselves in interactive workout scenarios, gamified training simulations, and virtual coaching sessions that enhance motivation, engagement, and enjoyment of fitness activities.

Strategies for Fitness Businesses to Adopt and Leverage AI Technologies

In "AI-Enhanced Adaptive Workout Programs: Revolutionizing Fitness," strategies for fitness businesses to adopt and leverage AI technologies are essential for staying competitive, driving innovation, and delivering value to customers in the rapidly evolving fitness landscape. Here are key strategies for fitness businesses to consider:

Invest in AI Talent and Expertise:

Fitness businesses should prioritize hiring or partnering with AI experts, data scientists, and machine learning engineers to build robust AI capabilities internally or externally. By investing in AI talent and expertise, fitness businesses can develop cutting-edge algorithms, predictive models, and data-driven insights that enhance the effectiveness and personalization of their workout programs.

Collect and Analyze User Data Effectively:

Fitness businesses should leverage AI technologies to collect and analyze user data effectively, including biometric measurements, workout history, performance metrics, and user feedback. By harnessing the power of AI-driven analytics, fitness businesses can gain valuable insights into user behavior, preferences, and trends, enabling them to tailor workouts, optimize training outcomes, and deliver personalized recommendations that resonate with their target audience.

Implement Personalized Workout Programs:

Fitness businesses should integrate AI technologies to develop personalized workout programs that cater to individual needs, goals, and fitness levels. By leveraging AI algorithms to analyze user data and preferences, fitness businesses can design customized exercise regimens, nutrition plans, and recovery strategies that maximize engagement, motivation, and results for their clients.

Enhance User Engagement and Retention:

Fitness businesses should use AI technologies to enhance user engagement and retention by offering interactive features, gamification elements, and social incentives that motivate and inspire users to stay active and committed to their fitness goals. By creating immersive workout experiences and fostering a sense of community and accountability, fitness businesses can build loyalty and trust among their customer base.

Integrate AI with Wearable Technology:
Fitness businesses should explore opportunities to integrate AI technologies with wearable devices and fitness trackers to track performance metrics, monitor biometric data, and provide real-time feedback to users during workouts. By harnessing the capabilities of wearable technology and AI-driven analytics, fitness businesses can empower users to optimize their training outcomes and achieve their fitness goals with precision and accuracy.

Offer Virtual Coaching and Personalization:
Fitness businesses should leverage AI technologies to offer virtual coaching and personalized guidance to users, providing them with real-time feedback, form correction tips, and motivational support throughout their fitness journey. By incorporating AI-driven chatbots, virtual assistants, and interactive coaching platforms, fitness businesses can scale their coaching services, expand their

reach, and deliver consistent, high-quality support to users wherever they are.

Ensure Data Privacy and Security:

Fitness businesses should prioritize data privacy and security by implementing robust encryption protocols, access controls, and data anonymization techniques to protect user information from unauthorized access, breaches, and misuse. By adhering to stringent data protection regulations and ethical guidelines, fitness businesses can build trust and credibility with their customers and stakeholders.

In conclusion, adopting and leveraging AI technologies is essential for fitness businesses to stay competitive, drive innovation, and deliver value to their customers in the digital age. By investing in AI talent and expertise, collecting and analyzing user data effectively, implementing personalized workout programs, enhancing user engagement and retention, integrating AI with wearable technology, offering virtual coaching and personalization, and ensuring data privacy and security, fitness businesses can

harness the transformative power of AI to revolutionize the way individuals engage with exercise, health, and wellness.

CHAPTER 6

CONCLUSION

In "AI-Enhanced Adaptive Workout Programs: Revolutionizing Fitness," we have explored the transformative potential of artificial intelligence (AI) in revolutionizing the fitness industry. Through an in-depth examination of AI-driven technologies, personalized workout programs, and innovative approaches to exercise and wellness, it is evident that AI is reshaping the way individuals engage with fitness, health, and well-being.

As we conclude our journey through the intersection of AI and fitness, several key insights emerge:

Personalization and Precision: AI enables the creation of highly personalized workout programs tailored to individual needs, preferences, and goals. By analyzing user data, biometrics, and performance metrics, AI algorithms optimize training outcomes and enhance the effectiveness of exercise regimens with unprecedented precision.

Engagement and Motivation: AI-driven fitness solutions foster greater engagement and motivation among users through interactive features, gamification elements, and social incentives. By creating immersive workout experiences and fostering a sense of community and accountability, AI enhances user adherence and commitment to their fitness journey.

Innovation and Accessibility: AI-driven innovations, such as virtual reality (VR), augmented reality (AR), and wearable technology, expand access to fitness resources and create new opportunities for engagement and participation. As technology evolves and becomes more accessible, individuals of all backgrounds and abilities can pursue healthier, more active lifestyles with greater convenience and flexibility.

Ethical Considerations and Data Privacy: As we embrace the benefits of AI in fitness, we must also address ethical considerations and data privacy concerns to ensure responsible use and deployment of technology. Safeguarding user privacy, transparency in data practices, and ethical use of AI algorithms are paramount to building trust and fostering a culture of accountability and integrity in the fitness industry.

Collaboration and Innovation: The future of AI-enhanced fitness lies in collaboration, innovation, and continuous learning. By fostering interdisciplinary collaboration, embracing emerging technologies, and embracing a culture of experimentation and agility, we can unlock new possibilities and drive positive change in the way individuals engage with exercise and wellness.

As we look ahead, the potential of AI-enhanced adaptive workout programs to revolutionize fitness is boundless. By harnessing the power of technology to optimize training outcomes, enhance user engagement, and promote holistic well-being, we can empower individuals to lead healthier, more fulfilling lives and unlock their full potential in pursuit of their fitness goals.

Summary of Key Insights and Findings

In "AI-Enhanced Adaptive Workout Programs: Revolutionizing Fitness," a comprehensive exploration of the intersection between artificial intelligence (AI) and fitness reveals transformative insights and findings that reshape the way individuals approach exercise, health, and well-being. Here's a summary of the key insights and findings from the book:

Personalization and Precision: AI-driven fitness solutions enable personalized workout programs tailored to individual needs, preferences, and goals. By analyzing user data, biometrics, and performance metrics, AI algorithms optimize training outcomes with unprecedented precision, enhancing the effectiveness and relevance of exercise regimens.

Engagement and Motivation: AI enhances user engagement and motivation through interactive features, gamification elements, and social incentives. By creating immersive workout experiences

and fostering a sense of community and accountability, AI-driven fitness platforms inspire greater adherence and commitment to fitness goals.

Innovation and Accessibility: AI-driven innovations, such as virtual reality (VR), augmented reality (AR), and wearable technology, expand access to fitness resources and create new opportunities for engagement and participation. Technology evolves to become more accessible, enabling individuals of all backgrounds and abilities to pursue healthier, more active lifestyles with greater convenience and flexibility.

Ethical Considerations and Data Privacy: The responsible use and deployment of AI in fitness require addressing ethical considerations and data privacy concerns. Safeguarding user privacy, transparency in data practices, and ethical use of AI algorithms are essential to building trust and fostering accountability and integrity in the fitness industry.

Collaboration and Innovation: The future of AI-enhanced fitness lies in collaboration, innovation, and continuous learning. Fostering interdisciplinary collaboration, embracing emerging technologies, and cultivating a culture of experimentation and agility unlock new possibilities and drive positive change in the fitness landscape.

Empowerment and Well-being: AI-enhanced adaptive workout programs empower individuals to lead healthier, more fulfilling lives by unlocking their full potential in pursuit of their fitness goals. By harnessing the power of technology to optimize training outcomes, enhance user engagement, and promote holistic well-being, individuals can achieve sustainable lifestyle changes and improve their quality of life.

Reflection on the Transformative Potential of AI in Fitness

In "AI-Enhanced Adaptive Workout Programs: Revolutionizing Fitness," the exploration of the transformative potential of artificial intelligence (AI) in fitness unveils a landscape defined by innovation, empowerment, and holistic well-being. Reflecting on the insights and revelations gleaned from the book, it becomes evident that AI has the power to revolutionize the way individuals engage with exercise, health, and fitness in profound ways.

The transformative potential of AI in fitness lies in its ability to personalize, optimize, and enhance the fitness experience for individuals of all backgrounds and abilities. Through advanced algorithms, data analytics, and machine learning techniques, AI-driven fitness solutions empower users to tailor their workouts, track their progress, and achieve their fitness goals with unprecedented precision and insight. By analyzing user data, biometrics, and performance metrics, AI algorithms optimize training outcomes, minimize the risk of injury, and inspire greater adherence and commitment to fitness goals.

Moreover, AI fosters a culture of innovation, collaboration, and continuous improvement within the fitness industry. By embracing emerging technologies, leveraging interdisciplinary expertise, and cultivating a culture of experimentation and agility, fitness professionals and businesses can unlock new possibilities and drive positive change in the way individuals approach exercise and wellness. From virtual reality (VR) and augmented reality (AR) experiences to wearable technology and personalized nutrition solutions, the integration of AI into fitness programming expands access to resources, enhances user engagement, and promotes holistic well-being on a global scale.

However, as we embark on this transformative journey, it is essential to address ethical considerations and data privacy concerns associated with the use of AI in fitness. Safeguarding user privacy, transparency in data practices, and ethical use of AI algorithms are paramount to building trust and fostering accountability and integrity in the fitness industry. By upholding ethical standards and regulatory compliance, fitness professionals and businesses can mitigate risks, protect user rights, and promote responsible innovation in the AI-driven fitness landscape.

Closing Thoughts on the Future Direction of the Industry and Opportunities for Innovation

As we conclude our exploration of "AI-Enhanced Adaptive Workout Programs: Revolutionizing Fitness," it is evident that the future direction of the fitness industry is poised for unprecedented transformation and innovation. The integration of artificial intelligence (AI) into fitness programming represents a paradigm shift in the way individuals engage with exercise, health, and wellness, unlocking new possibilities and opportunities for growth in the digital age.

Looking ahead, several key trends and opportunities emerge that will shape the future direction of the industry and drive innovation in AI-enhanced fitness:

Personalization and Precision:

The future of fitness lies in personalized, data-driven experiences that cater to individual needs, preferences, and goals. By leveraging AI algorithms to analyze user data, track performance metrics, and deliver tailored recommendations, fitness professionals and businesses can optimize training outcomes, enhance user engagement, and promote long-term adherence to fitness goals.

Integration of Emerging Technologies: The convergence of AI with emerging technologies, such as virtual reality (VR), augmented reality (AR), and wearable technology, will redefine the fitness experience and expand access to resources and engagement opportunities. By embracing these technologies, fitness professionals can create immersive workout experiences, gamified training simulations, and interactive coaching platforms that inspire greater motivation, enjoyment, and participation among users.

Expansion into Corporate Wellness and Healthcare: The integration of AI-driven fitness solutions into corporate wellness programs and healthcare initiatives presents new opportunities for collaboration and innovation. By partnering with employers, insurers, and healthcare providers, fitness professionals can develop scalable, data-driven solutions that promote employee health, reduce healthcare costs, and improve population health outcomes.

Ethical Considerations and Data Privacy:

As AI technologies continue to evolve and permeate every aspect of the fitness industry, it is essential to prioritize ethical considerations and data privacy concerns. Safeguarding user privacy, transparency in data practices, and ethical use of AI algorithms are paramount to building trust and fostering accountability and integrity in the AI-driven fitness landscape.

Continuous Learning and Adaptation:

The future direction of the fitness industry requires a commitment to continuous learning, adaptation, and innovation. By staying abreast of emerging trends, evolving consumer preferences, and technological advancements, fitness professionals and businesses can remain agile, responsive, and relevant in a rapidly changing market landscape.

9 798883 530851